WAITING FOR A NEW HIP?

Tips to make your wait easier

MR JONATHAN HULL MD FRCS(ORTH)
CONSULTANT ORTHOPAEDIC SURGEON
(also waiting)

First published 2023 by Magic Daisy Publishing
Printed through Amazon

www.magicdaisypublishing.co.uk

Copyright © Magic Daisy Publishing 2023
Text copyright © Jonathan Hull 2023

The moral rights of the author have been asserted

ISBN   979-8-3767-0162-1

Printed and bound by Amazon

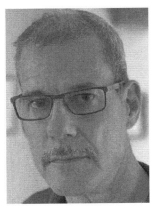

Jonathan was educated at Uppingham School and Birmingham University Medical School, graduating in 1983. He joined the Army in 1980 and served for 19 years with postings to Germany and the USA and operational tours in Northern Ireland, Iraq, Congo, Bosnia and Kosovo. He was parachute trained and provided surgical support for UK Special Forces.

After leaving the Army he was a Consultant Orthopaedic Surgeon at Frimley Park Hospital from 1999-2020, specialising in all aspects of hip surgery as well as trauma management.

Jonathan is married and has four grown-up children and two grandchildren. He has now retired from NHS practice and lives in Norfolk where, as it happens, he grew up. He shoots regularly at Bisley and has represented Hampshire, England and Great Britain; his shooting is on hold at the moment as he can't lie flat on his front because of his hip.

He injured his right hip parachuting in 1996. Eventually he reluctantly accepted it needed sorting out and he underwent a hip replacement in November 2021.

Now his left hip is playing up ...

PREFACE

If you have already read *Hip Expectations*, you may be in the fortunate position of having had your replacement by now, in which case I doubt you will have bought this book. I hope it went well and you are pleased with the outcome.

You may, however, be in the same place as I am at the moment and are wondering if you actually need the other one doing as well. Only around 10% of people ever need their other hip replacing once the first has been done, and even if the second one was a little arthritic all along, it may not progress very much or require replacement. But mine does, and I am trying to live with it for a while.

I thought it may be helpful to provide some advice and guidance about doing just that, with my own experience as a baseline, and as I am writing it whilst I am waiting, it may be more helpful and accurate than if I delay it until afterwards. And it gives me something to be doing whilst I am becoming increasingly lame!

Fiona Goult, physio extraordinaire, has already done considerable work on helping patients prepare for hip replacement as well as successfully guiding their rehab afterwards. Her input to the exercise section in particular is really helpful.

With the current state of NHS waiting lists, you may be in real trouble with your hip and cannot see when it is ever going to be done. Please don't despair as this difficult time will eventually pass; hopefully some of what we say will be helpful while you patiently endure your pain and stiffness.

INDEX

INTRODUCTION

'BUT YOU DON'T HAVE TO WAIT' I hear you say. 'You're a surgeon and can get your hip done when you want'.

That's true, and when I decided I'd had enough of my first hip, I was indeed able to arrange my replacement for more or less when I wanted it. If you have worked in a hospital for 25 years and have trained the surgeon who is going to do it, I'll admit it is not difficult to make things happen.

I am now in the position where I have fully recovered from the right hip replacement a year ago, and my left, which was of trivial concern then, has now progressed and I am clearly going to need a matching pair before too long.

'So, why the wait?', you ask.

The thing is, I have decided to fully retire at the end of 2024. There is a process called 'Revalidation' for doctors, and the General Medical Council requires us all to be assessed every five years to ensure we are competent and safe to continue to practise. That is all well and good and an important safety issue, but it involves a significant amount of hoop-jumping and endless forms, 360-degree appraisals and many other tiresome chores. My next revalidation date is November 2024, and I have decided that will be the right time for me to put away my scalpel for good. I would much prefer that people ask '*why* are you retiring?', rather than '*when* are you retiring?', if you see what I mean.

So, instead of taking three months off to have my left hip replaced now or in the next two years, I am minded to make my next hip replacement the very last thing I do at my place of work.

Hence the wait.

WHY ARE *YOU* WAITING?

If you are reading this to while away the time as you wait patiently on an NHS list, becoming increasingly depressed at the newspaper reports of 7 million people currently waiting for routine surgery such as joint replacement, then you are probably in the largest group of people for whom I have written it.

The NHS was just about coping prior to the Coronavirus Pandemic in 2020, but the necessary suspension of routine operations during the various lockdowns to protect NHS capacity and help reduce viral transmission, together with the currently increased demand due to delayed presentation as people avoided troubling their GPs during the Covid-19 period, has created a massive increase in numbers of patients now needing surgery.

To be fair, there have always been waiting lists. Back in the heady days of the Millennium, when Prime Minister Tony Blair was informed that patients were waiting up to 18 months for hip and knee replacement, he supposedly said words to the effect of:

"18 months? - I want that down to 18 weeks as soon as possible!"

And so it was that '18 weeks' became the mantra and the absolute target we all strived for right through until 2020. We didn't always achieve it, and some areas were better than others, but various schemes were created to offer patients surgery in areas of the country that were less busy, to get the majority in within at least one year and for Trusts, long waiters were always a priority.

Going further back, when I was a very young doctor, 2-year waits were not unusual and were generally well-tolerated. It was commonplace for patients to be referred to orthopaedics long before they were actually suitable for surgery, to get onto the list early, so that when their turn came around, they were ready. I suspect that ploy may have started to creep back now.

Of course, there are other reasons why patients are waiting. For some, there may be medical reasons why a hip replacement is not suitable at the moment. Maybe a heart condition or other medical problem needs treating first? Perhaps the patient is very overweight and it would be dangerous to undergo surgery? Hopefully most of these medical reasons can be sorted out and sadly for a very few, surgery may never be an option.

It may not be just medical. Consider the patient in their late 50's who plans to retire at 60. He or she may be in a job that they cannot just up and leave for 8-12 weeks to recover from a replacement and for them, the wait is preferable to disruption to their job and potential livelihood or pension.

Or, the professional sportsman/sportswoman with an arthritic hip that is preventing them continuing with their vigorous activity. They may be advised that hip replacement is their only surgical option but that this would not allow them to return to their sport. Faced with that, some will choose to wait and reduce their activities. Some may opt for surgery and try to continue. There is a well-known professional tennis player who continues to compete at the highest level after having a hip resurfacing - but no-one can know for how long.

Then there is the waiter with insight. Someone who has already been through a replacement, knows exactly what it entails, and can therefore make an informed decision about when it is time to get the other side done. They may be strongly influenced by their experience – if it went well and they recovered quickly with no problems then they are likely to have a lower threshold for calling time on the second side. If, on the other hand, it was not such a positive experience and they struggled to recover, the opposite may be true. I would say that the majority of knee replacement patients will take their time going back for the other side – they know just how hard the recovery can be.

Whatever the reason, someone with a hip that is bad enough to warrant replacement is going to be having symptoms and these will be predominantly:

PAIN and STIFFNESS.

The remainder of this book will concentrate on how best to cope with these and their associated problems.

EFFECTS OF WAITING

As a general principle, in the medical world if you discover a problem, you try and resolve it without delay. You diagnose an infection, you give antibiotics. The patient has diabetes, you give them insulin. A broken bone - you fix it.

In an ideal world, an Elysium, everyone would enjoy perfect health and if this was threatened, a magical scanner would restore it immediately.

Focussing on the arthritic hip joint, the normal pattern is that the patient slowly develops pain and stiffness over several months or years. They present to their GP, and after a confirmatory x-ray, they are informed that they have arthritis and will need to be seen by an orthopaedic surgeon for consideration for a replacement. An alternative pathway is that they are injured after a fall or a traffic collision perhaps, and it is found that the hip joint is fractured for which a replacement would be the preferred treatment. It is not always quite that simple but for the purposes of this section, let's just say it is.

In either scenario, waiting is involved. In the first, there may be a considerable wait prior to diagnosis. Hip pain is usually slow to develop over a long period. A slight niggle after exercise, a 'groin strain', a dull ache after a long walk, are all common initial symptoms. They are intermittent and it often takes a considerable time for one to acknowledge there might be a problem. Eventually the good days are outnumbered by the bad and, with or without encouragement from other halves or family, the patient goes on to seek help.

For the injury scenario above, the only wait is in A&E, and hopefully that will not be as extended as it is at present, by the time you are reading this.

After diagnosis, and this is generally by x-ray although sometimes an MRI may be needed, then the proper waiting starts.   It may be agreed that the hip is only mildly arthritic, and that you will need to wait for it to become worse before considering operative treatment.   In the meantime, lose weight, take painkillers, do physio etc.

Or it may be severe.   Somehow arthritis has developed without you really being aware of it and now the hip joint is very diseased, and replacement is the only option.

Reality is probably somewhere in between and wherever you are on that spectrum, it is likely that at some point you will be told it is time for you to go onto a waiting list. If you are seeing a surgeon privately, then that list may be very short, and you are offered a date immediately. If on the NHS, then you may be given no firm date but are told that the average wait time is approximately xx months, although that may be subject to change.

Knowing for certain that the hip is ready for replacement, and seeing your x-rays for real, does seem to make it more painful for some reason. I had exactly that and, until I had my first x-ray, I was able to convince myself it really wasn't that bad. Being told you need a replacement is quite likely to make it feel worse but don't worry, it isn't suddenly any different just because you know about it, and it won't suddenly deteriorate either.

Sleep issues

Disturbed sleep caused by a painful hip is a common problem for many patients who are waiting, myself included. Usually, getting to sleep when one is tired is not too difficult but staying asleep can be. It is not unusual to wake up with discomfort after a few hours and then not be able to get back off again; if you lie on the bad side, it hurts due to pressure and if you lie on the other side, the bad hip pulls and aches. Placing a pillow between your knees can certainly reduce this pulling and often makes it more comfortable. There are specially shaped foam knee pillows designed to be placed between the knees, and these can certainly help (as long as you can find a way to keep them in position!)

It it worth experimenting with alternatives to your normal bed during this period, and clearly if your mattress is due replacement, now is a good time. Firmer mattresses tend to be good for bad backs, not so much for painful hips, but a soft mattress may not suit your partner. Many patients tell me they are only able to sleep lying on their backs, but this does tend to make you snore, and we all know how that can lead to marital stress!

It is not unusual for patients to tell me they can only sleep in an armchair and although this not ideal, a few good hours in a chair is vastly preferable to poor and disturbed dozing in your bed. If you can get comfortable in an armchair, perhaps with your legs out on a stool or cushion, or on a sofa maybe, and you can regularly get back to sleep this way, then my advice is don't fight it. It won't be for ever and any sleep is better than no sleep.

You'll have to work it out for yourself, and everyone is different, but my message is to be flexible and don't rule out a temporary sleeping location just for the period you are waiting.

Needless to say, it is useful to take pain medication to increase your chance of getting a decent sleep and timing your last tablets for 30-60 minutes before you retire to bed makes good sense.

Hips usually take months or years to become significantly worse, and I have many patients on my list who I see annually with very mild progression. Please don't despair that while you are on the waiting list you will end up in a wheelchair, never to walk again.

You won't.

MEDICATION

Pain is neither pleasant nor useful, except perhaps to stop one overdoing it. Chronic, unrelenting pain is demoralising and depressing, making everything difficult and miserable.

That said, hip pain is usually only really unpleasant when you try to do too much and generally can be controlled with medium strength analgesia and sensible behaviour.

The trick is knowing your limits, and there everyone is different. I have had patients who are distressed that they cannot manage their daily 5 km run and want me to make that possible. For them, the prospect of not running is unacceptable and they want to know what can be done to resolve that. I was in the Army for 19 years and I know all about running, was actually quite good at it, but I have to say I don't consider it is one of life's essential activities. In the film Forest Gump, the lead character summed it up after he had run from Alabama to the West coast of America with the words: 'I'm pretty tired...I think I'll go home now', and that was it, no more running for him. I get that.

However, having a stiff and painful hip is very annoying. As well as not being able to run, assuming you wish to, all sorts of everyday things are difficult. Cutting your toenails is a struggle (tip: sit on the penultimate stair immediately after a bath or shower and put your foot on the bottom stair – works for me). Having to kneel down to pick something up off the floor. Needing to use a shoehorn, even with slip-ons. Going up the stairs leading with your good leg for every step. And so on.

None of which are dreadful or life-changing, but they are so irritating and make you feel, well, just old.

Simple painkillers can make a huge difference and can really reduce that irritation, or at least make you less conscious of your limitations.

Paracetamol

I really like this. It's safe, it's cheap as chips (cheaper actually) and it really does work. But – you must take it very regularly. Two x 500mg tablets or capsules EVERY FOUR HOURS. Not every six or eight hours, every four. The maximum recommended daily dose is 8 tabs/caps so it may be worth delaying the last two of the day until just before bedtime, eg. two at 08.00, 12.00, 16.00, 21.00, or whatever suits you. I set my phone to alarm four hours after I take my two paracetamols, all through the day, to remind me. If I don't, I forget, (which is a sure sign that they are working), but then the effect is diminished. If you go six or eight hours between doses, it doesn't work as well and you are always playing catch-up.

I really don't think it matters whether you take the cheapest supermarket brand at 29p (currently) for 16 tabs or fancy glossy Panadol Extra costing £3 a packet, as they seem to be just as effective (believe me, I've tried them all). Adding caffeine and/or aspirin is no better as far as I'm concerned, and you may find they upset your stomach, as I have discovered.

Key message: Every four hours. On the dot.

Just like orthopaedic surgeons – simple but effective.

Anti-inflammatories

These are a different class of drug to simple painkillers and can be taken alongside them without causing problems. Sometimes referred to as NSAIDs (non-steroidal anti-inflammatory drugs), the best known is Ibuprofen or Nurofen and you can buy these over the counter as 200mg capsules or tablets. The recommended dose is 400mg (two tabs), every eight hours and they need to be taken regularly as well if they are going to work. I have nothing particularly against ibuprofen and some patients tell me it helps, but it does come with side effects. Heartburn, or gastritis, is not uncommon and if you are asthmatic, they are not recommended as they may cause an attack. Also, if you have any problems with your kidneys, ibuprofen can make these worse and it should be avoided.

And for me, they just don't seem to work.

There are stronger NSAIDs available on prescription, namely Naproxen and Diclofenac. Your GP would need to give you a prescription for these and will know if they are not suitable for you. Again, they do seem to help, and many patients tell me they work for them, but they need to be taken regularly and continuously to be effective. It can take up to three or four days to see a difference.

COX-2 inhibitors

These are a more advanced generation of anti-inflammatory and for me, they are the most effective. The big advantage, other than the fact that they work, is that they only need to be taken once a day as they have a long half-life. It is so much easier to remember to take them, either with your first cup of tea in the morning or last thing at night. It doesn't matter when you take them as long as it is the same every day, and they also take a few days to 'kick in'.

My preference is Etoricoxib 60mg daily but other Cox-2 inhibitors available are Meloxicam and Celebrex. They have a lower risk of gastritis, but if you do get that, you may need to take Omeprazole (Nexium) as well to protect your stomach lining. Again, they are not recommended for those with asthma or kidney problems. The other issue is cost. They are more expensive than ibuprofen and naproxen but the cost has actually fallen considerably in the past few years. Your GP may say they are not permitted to prescribe them on the NHS but you could request a private prescription. You will have to pay the pharmacy for the drugs, but I can tell you that 56 tabs of Etoricoxib 60mg now costs me around £9 – that works out at 16p per day. Well worth it in my opinion.

On a personal note, I had been taking Etoricoxib for a couple of years prior my hip replacement last year and I stopped it one week pre-op as instructed – within 2 days I was in real trouble. It works.

Stronger stuff

Probably the most effective painkiller available is **Diamorphine**. We used to give this to patients with an acute heart attack, but I doubt they do now. Clearly this is not appropriate for hip pain, and you would become addicted in no time. There are several other opiate-like drugs on the market with less strength and less risk of addiction, with names like **Codeine, Oramorph, Tramadol, Fentanyl** etc. My own view is to try and avoid them if at all possible. All have potential side-effects (constipation, nausea, drowsiness, addiction, tolerance) and I don't think that they do much more than blunt your senses in the long term.

I am no expert in pain management and the above is my opinion based on both years of speaking to my patients and my own experience with my hips.

> Other than for what you can buy over the counter, you **must** discuss pain medication with your GP or specialist to ensure that whatever you take will not harm you.

Homeopathy

I am not qualified to offer you a balanced discussion concerning alternative medicines. I am also not so prehistoric to argue that none have any value for patients. Doctors do tend to be a bit sniffy about treatments that may not have been fully evaluated or be approved by bodies such as the National Institute for Health and Care Excellence (NICE), but numerous patients have told me over the years that various products such as fish oils, glucosamine, vitamins, supplements etc have worked for them.

Acupuncture can also help and for some it is a really effective way of controlling pain. I have no idea how it works but that doesn't matter, as long as it does.

And if any benefit is just due to the placebo effect, so what? It's still a benefit, and 'every little helps' (as that supermarket is always telling us).

ACTIVITY & EXERCISE

This is arguably the most important section of this book. Getting the correct balance between the right level of activity and appropriate rest, is vital to managing your hip while you are waiting. Everyone is different and no two people have exactly the same body shape, expectations, demands and pain threshold but I will try and set out what I consider to be the general principles and what I use to guide my activity during this tiresome period of my life.

Shape

By which I mean your weight, or BMI. The force transmitted through our joints is proportional to our weight and for the hip, the joint reaction force may be 2-3 times body weight when climbing stairs or running. If your hip is already damaged by arthritis, then it is not moving in the normal frictionless manner and will react badly to increased force, hence the increased pain on attempting high impact activity such as jogging, or badminton etc.

A patient once told me they only had significant pain when they carried a full shopping bag. It would therefore seem logical that losing the equivalent weight, say 4-5 kg, should reduce pain for some patients. And it really does. Time and time again, I am told that losing weight has helped and unless you are particularly underweight, I would always suggest you try – even just a little can really make a difference.

The converse is definitely true, and every effort should be made to keep your weight at least steady. I know, I know, you can't exercise properly because of your hip and for some, regular exercise is the mainstay of their efforts to keep their weight down. I sympathise completely and do understand.

The alternative is to adapt your diet. That's easy to say and hard to do, but the science of it is irrefutable. Less fuel in, less excess to store, less weight to carry.

I like my food as much as anyone else and I have a cooked breakfast every single day. I'm lucky in that I can eat three good meals and not put on weight. There is plenty of help out there whether it be diet plans, weight loss groups, dieticians, nutritionalists and the like, or just plain old common sense and will-power (without some of which the others are likely to fail to be honest).

The fact is, if you want to have less pain while you're waiting for your hip,

- and you would like the operation to be technically easier for your surgeon,

- and you would like to have an easier recovery,

- and you would like to feel fitter and healthier...

...you know what to do.

   'That's all I have to say about that' – Forest Gump (again)

Activity

Here I mean regular daily activity, not exercise per se. The sort of things one takes for granted like bathing, dressing, walking to the shops, sitting at your desk at work, catching the train, driving the car and so on. All these mundane activities may eventually come to be affected by your bad hip and you may need to moderate or change what you do to accommodate it.

When I am talking to a patient about the optimal time for surgery, a phrase I often use is: 'Don't back yourself into a chair' by which I mean don't put up with increasing symptoms to the point where all you do all day is sit and watch the world go by. You (we) must remain active as much as possible but at the same time try and avoid things that will be especially painful.

Example: driving my wife's car is not only uncomfortable, but makes my hip hurt for a while after a journey. Solution: drive mine. That's a simple one but they all count.

Another: weeding the garden. I can do it by squatting down but it's so much more comfortable using a kneeler. It takes longer and is more awkward but at the end of the afternoon, it hurts less.

Avoidance of pain is good providing you remain active and busy. Everyone needs to work it out for themselves, and compromises are fine. No-one wants to use a walking stick, but a walking *pole*? – that's fine because proper walkers use those don't they?

No pain = no pain. ('No pain, no gain' is <u>definitely</u> not appropriate)

Remaining active will also help promote good circulation which helps prevent venous thrombosis, or DVT, and may reduce the risk of this after your replacement too.

Exercise

It is important to cover exercise of the affected hip and also general exercise of the whole body. The latter may involve the hip as well, but specific exercises to maintain the hip and its surrounding soft tissues, are essential.

Hip work

The hip is a ball and socket joint and normally moves very freely in all three dimensions. As arthritis progresses, and the joint surface breaks down, the range of motion tends to reduce and as a result, the hip capsule stiffens and tightens up. It also becomes thicker and less supple, adding to the stiffness.

If you do nothing at all with the hip, for example retire to your bed and completely immobilise the joint, it may become stiffer and stiffer, to the point where it will not move at all. This can occasionally be seen in patients in a coma and the changes in the joint may be irreversible.

In reality, of course there will always be some motion, and forward flexion in particular is maintained just by sitting and walking, to the extent that the hip can become a virtual hinge joint, only moving in the frontal plane. This is clearly not ideal, and some rotation is necessary to allow even relatively normal function.

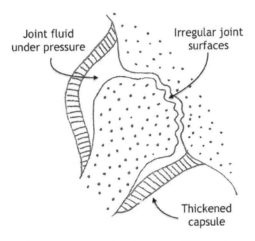

Three reasons for increased hip pain, stiffness and reduced movement

The other main issue with hip arthritis is progressive tightening and shortening of the hip flexor tendon, psoas, which blends with the front of the hip capsule. As psoas tightens, the hip fails to fully straighten when you stand, and this is responsible for the characteristic stoop that many hip patients develop. It is as though there is a tight elastic band over the front of the hip, and this stops you standing fully upright.

These effects can be mitigated to an extent by exercise, and maintaining even a reduced range of motion is very helpful. We would recommend the following on at least a daily basis:

Buttock squeeze Lie on your back, head and neck supported by a pillow. Squeeze your buttocks and hold. Reps x10 Hold 5 seconds Sets 2-3 x a day	
Lying on your back, tighten the muscles of your front thigh. Pull your toes towards you, bend your ankles and push your knees down firmly against the bed. Hold for 5 seconds. Reps x10. Sets 2-3 x a day	
Lying on your back, bend your bad leg by sliding the heel up towards you. If it is not too painful, you can then gently let your knee fall out sideways as far as it will comfortably go, bringing it slowly back to the midline before lowering it. Reps x10 Sets 2-3 x a day	

In standing, squeeze your buttocks and bring one leg back behind you, keeping your knee straight. Do not lean forwards or let your lower back arch. Hold onto a work surface or chair for support. Reps x10 Sets 2-3x a day	
Bend the knee and lift your foot off the floor and hold. Try and get the knee up to waist level if you can. Reps x 10 Sets 2-3 x a day	
Lift your leg sideways. Hold onto a work surface or chair for support. Try not to lean sideways as you lift the leg to the side. Reps x10 Sets 2-3x a day	
Lying on your good side, clench your buttocks and lift the bad leg upwards, keeping the knee locked out straight. Try and hold it up for 5 seconds and gently lower. Reps x10 Sets 2-3 x day	

Flex down slowly into a squat position. Hold onto a work surface or chair for support, (have a chair positioned behind you for safety if you are worried about falling). Only go as far as you can rise up from. Reps x 10 Sets 2 a day	
With your feet firmly on floor, and your knees flexed to 90°, lift up your pelvis towards the ceiling. Try and hold this arch position for at least 20 seconds, thrusting your hips up as far as possible. You should feel the strain across the front of the hip, and this means the tight capsule is being stretched. Reps x 5 Sets 2 a day	

All the lying down exercises above can be done on your bed if getting to the floor is difficult.

If you find that any of these exercises cause symptoms that concern you, please seek some more personalised advice from your GP or a Chartered Physiotherapist.

General exercise

At the very least, try and go out for a walk everyday. It doesn't have to be very far, but if you can manage 20-30

27

minutes of brisk walking on the flat, so much the better. It is better to walk rather than amble, and if you can get a rhythm going it will be easier and more beneficial.

If you can, try and take full strides, as this will help stretch that tight capsule at the front of the hip. I would go as far as saying that if you can tolerate making it hurt a little in the groin, particularly as the other leg goes forwards, you are probably doing good and helping the capsule stretch. Don't overdo it though and only cause slight discomfort not real pain.

Walk tall if you can. Be aware of the tendency to stoop and to bend slightly at the waist and try and make yourself stand up as straight as you can. It is easy to forget this and slip back into stooping, so you will have to concentrate.

Sometimes counting can help, as can listening to music with a steady beat. You almost need to march, and you should try to make each pace the same length.

Keep to the flat and avoid uneven ground. Country walks are very pleasant but uneven ground may well cause you to tweak your hip; this can cause a little more swelling in the joint, which then makes it hurt more, get stiffer and offers no benefit at all.

Small slopes are fine but as soon as you start to have to lean forwards to get up a steep incline you will begin to stress the hip again and may make it hurt to no advantage. It's the same with stairs so don't be shy of using a lift if there is one.

Walking poles or a stick are good options if you feel you are limping. It is better to use a walking aid and walk correctly than not use them and limp. Remember to use a stick on the *opposite* side to your affected hip.

Low impact exercise

There is no reason to avoid the gym and if you have a routine visit to a spa or fitness centre, or you enjoy a regular exercise class, don't stop going. As long as you avoid high impact activities such as the running machines, you should do no harm at all. Having said that, walking on a treadmill may sometimes be more comfortable than walking outside for your daily walk as the treadmill has a certain degree of shock absorbency built in. The built-in handrails may also offer some support and that may minimise limping (and let's face it, the climate in the gym is also often more pleasant than the weather outside in the UK!) Cross-trainers are good, as are rowing machines due to the lack of impact involved. Don't worry on the rower if your leg excursion is limited somewhat due to the hip.

Work within the movement you have (and you may find over time your range of movement increases). If you use weights, then be sensible. Lots of light weight reps rather than maximal leg presses. Use the gym to help stretch the hip and maintain or improve muscle strength: it is ok to be guided by how it feels. Again, gentle stretches to mild discomfort are safe, but don't make your eyes water! The instructors in your gym should be on hand to help adjust your programme to suit your individual situation.

Don't forget to work your upper body muscle groups too while in the gym, or with light weights at home (a can of baked beans in each hand can be a good way to start if you haven't used weights before). When you do finally have the surgery, you will need those arms to be strong to use crutches post operatively and help you get in and out of chairs etc more easily.

Swimming

In an ideal world we would all have access to a warm swimming pool on a daily basis.   Public pools, with slippery floors and cold changing rooms can be less than inviting, but if you can go swimming it can only help.   Even just walking in a pool with the water at chest height can be very therapeutic and hip exercises supported by the water are easy and effective.

There seems to be a widespread concern about breaststroke for hip patients.   I would agree it is not advisable immediately post replacement but for those of you awaiting surgery, gentle attempts at this are definitely worth trying. Hip rotation, which is always restricted by arthritis, can be significantly improved by doing breaststroke and it is safe and well-supported by the water. A crawl kick is good for muscle strength. Try doing a few lengths or widths of swimming (if you can or want to swim) then doing a few exercises (see below) then a few more lengths/widths, then a few more exercises; mixing the swimming and exercises will probably make you less sore afterwards. Take it easy if this is all new to you, things tend to feel amazing while you are in the water, but the next day you may feel achy and sore, so introduce changes gradually.

Aqua-robics classes are also good and worth trying if you can. Exercising with other people can be beneficial as well.

Suggestions of exercises that can be done in a pool:

- Try to be chest deep in the water to be able to use the resistance of the water as well as the buoyancy.
- Walking forwards.
- Walking backwards.
- Walking sideways/ side steps.
- Mini squats.
- Mini lunges.
  (you may need to be in slightly shallower water for the last 2 exercises - please don't drown!)
- Float the knee up towards your chest and then push in back down to the floor of the pool. Repeat, then change legs so that each leg has a turn.

Examples of good and bad exercise types:

Good exercise	Bad exercise
Walking *(not uneven ground)*	Running / jogging
Swimming	Badminton, squash
Low-impact aerobics	High-impact aerobics
Rowing machine / cross-trainer	Mountaineering
Static bike or electric bike	
Pilates/ Yoga / Dancing	
Doubles tennis	

Even the activities in the 'Good' column above may need to be altered to suit your situation; with yoga and Pilates for example, there may be positions you can't get into due to your hip, but focus on the things you *can* do and maybe do more of those, rather than worrying about the things you *can't* do.

SAFETY CONCERNS

Can living with an arthritic hip ever be a safety concern? Not long ago I was looking forward to some quality time with my 3-year-old granddaughter whilst my wife took our grandson out for the afternoon. To my surprise my wife suggested we probably shouldn't go out for a walk as, if my granddaughter suddenly decided to run out into the road, I might not be able to move quickly enough to stop her.

I was really upset, but I knew she was right as I realised it was a risk and not something I could live with if it happened. Although I appear to be moving normally enough, I'm not sure I could react really quickly if I had to. Makes you think, doesn't it?

It is approaching Christmas as I write this and yesterday, I was putting up some lights on the outside of our house. Nothing too gaudy, just 500 icicle lights hanging from the gutter to massively outdo the neighbours and send our electricity bill through the roof – well, you've just got to, haven't you? Anyway, that involved going up a long ladder and after a couple of times, I realised that not only was it really quite painful, but my hip didn't feel that steady. I'm quite good with heights but I did worry that my hip might give way on me.

Which would have been awkward.

These are just two personal examples but I'm sure you will be able to think of other instances where your painful hip might be a liability.

Driving

After having a hip replacement there are some well-established guidelines for when it is time to resume driving, based principally on safety and comfort. You must be able to control the car and do an emergency stop, and you must be comfortable even if you get stuck in a traffic jam. For most people this is 6-8 weeks after a right hip and sooner for a left.

But what about before the operation? Certainly, you must be sure you are safe. The hip would have to be pretty bad to stop you driving for safety reasons, but comfort can be an issue, especially for long drives. Some cars are not ideal for a bad hip and getting in and out of a low car can be awkward and uncomfortable. You find yourself looking for parking spaces which have a clear space to the right, and tight multi-storeys can be a nightmare.

Tip: try and park right on the line, or just over it if you dare, to discourage anyone from taking that empty space to your right so that it's clear when you return to the car.

Other less anti-social advice might be to plan your journey to include frequent stops to stretch off, and to change the seat position regularly to try and prevent your hip getting stuck in one position.

Finally, do be careful crossing the road after you get out of the car - you may not be able to move quickly enough if you leave it too late.

RED FLAGS

The norm is for the hip to become progressively more uncomfortable and stiffer, as what is left of the joint surface disappears. Once all the cartilage has gone, and the joint is truly bone-on-bone, sometimes the process just stops and nothing much changes. You remain very stiff, and the range of motion is restricted to just forwards and backwards, with no rotation to speak of, but the pain may actually become less intrusive. I believe the pain one feels is mainly caused by inflammation and excess fluid production within the hip, and as this is under pressure as the hip cannot expand like the knee does, it will hurt. If the inflammation reduces, once the hip is just dry bone-on-bone, sometimes the pain whilst at rest does recede.

Increasing pain

Progressively increasing severe pain is not good and is the first of my Red Flags to discuss.

The head of the femur has a blood supply. This comes in at the base of the neck, through the capsule, and the bone is nourished by this and kept alive. If that blood supply is restricted or blocked altogether, the effect is that the bone dies inside.

THIS IS VERY PAINFUL.

The condition is called Avascular Necrosis (AVN) or Osteonecrosis. It is rare and can sometimes occur in a previously healthy hip, when sudden onset of pain can be hard to diagnose at first. Eventually x-rays and MRI scans will reveal the bony changes and whilst it may sometimes resolve spontaneously, it can lead to early hip replacement often in quite young patients.

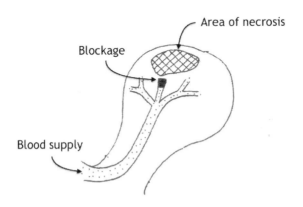

Avascular Necrosis - loss of blood supply
to a segment of the femoral head

A small proportion of patients with established osteoarthritis, possibly already on a waiting list, will develop AVN as well, to add insult to injury. They may have been hobbling along relatively well for months or even years when they experience a gradual but relentless increase in their pain. The pain is not controlled with simple medication and can render one almost immobile. It is not improved by sitting or lying down and definitely not by trying to exercise.

If you can get to an orthopaedic surgeon and the diagnosis is confirmed, most of us would try do the hip replacement on an urgent basis.

Locking

All arthritic hips are stiff. They are meant to be, and stiffness generally increases slowly and insidiously over a long period. You gradually find it harder to reach your toes, put on your socks, get into the car etc and although you compensate by using your lower back to bend forwards, eventually you find you have to kneel down to pick something up off the floor and so on.

But, if your hip suddenly stops moving, that may be a problem. Locking up of the hip can be caused by a number of things. The cartilage rim around the socket can get jammed between the head and the cup, although in advanced arthritis this rim has usually disappeared. Part of the bone at the edge of the socket or the head can break off and get stuck. This bone is called osteophyte and forms as a result of the arthritis. It is not particularly strong, and pieces can separate from time to time. If they become jammed in the joint, it can lock up and be stuck more or less completely.

The effect can be sudden, and the hip just seizes up. If you are sitting down, you can't get the leg to go straight when you stand, and if you are standing or walking, the hip might suddenly collapse and make you fall.

Again, unless this locking sorts itself out quickly, there is little choice but for you to go to A&E, by ambulance if necessary, as it is not feasible to just sit around for days and, as well as being stuck, the hip is likely to be very painful.

It is certainly worth trying to get things moving by gently moving the leg backwards forwards and sideways, maybe with someone else helping to move it for you passively, but not if it is agony and too painful to endure. If after 30-60 minutes it is not improving, call 999.

Progressive stiffness

Yes of course your hip is stiff, and some days are better than others but if you find the joint becomes steadily much stiffer and more immobile, either with or without more pain, then there is the possibility that the femoral head may have collapsed on itself, particularly if the pain is really noticeable. This is not common, but we do see it from time to time. For surgeons it is an indication that we need to operate soon, and the patient will usually be moved into the urgent category. As the head collapses the rest of the joint tightens up and it can make the operation more difficult and the result less predictable.

If you do find the hip becomes much stiffer, without respite, I would advise that you contact your GP and request a new x-ray as soon as possible.

Sepsis

It is very rare for an arthritic hip to develop infection, almost unheard of, but there is one structure close to the hip that occasionally does cause trouble.

The hip flexor tendon, psoas, runs from just below the hip joint, through the pelvis and attaches to the lower segments of the lumbar spine. As it traverses the pelvis and abdomen, it can be vulnerable to spread of infection from either the spine (e.g., infected intervertebral disc) or in the abdomen (e.g., diverticular abscess).

A psoas abscess means infected fluid collects in the sheath around the tendon and this may produce a warm swelling in the groin as well as increased pain. The hip can go into spasm and lock up and the infection may cause you to feel most unwell with fevers, flushes and hot sweats or shivering.

This is an emergency and needs to be diagnosed and treated urgently, via A&E if no other help is available.

I had a patient with this recently and it was not immediately obvious (to me), but fortunately the GP recognised that the patient was unwell and did the appropriate blood tests. That patient needed several weeks of intravenous antibiotics, and I am happy to say that they have now had a successful hip replacement.

I must stress that the vast majority of hip patients on the waiting list WILL NOT develop one of the above problems and will proceed on to have their replacement without an issue.

TIPS AND TRICKS

Everyone needs to work out what to do for themselves to try and make life just a little easier. Whether it is to bath or shower, to sit on the stairs to cut your toenails or come downstairs backwards. We cannot possibly cover everything but hopefully the following will be of some help:

Chairs	You may need to avoid deep armchairs and sofas as they can be difficult to get out of. Higher chairs with arms to push on are better and easier and try and lean forwards with your chest as you start to rise up. The same applies on the loo when you are ready to stand up.
Stairs	'Good leg to Heaven, Bad leg to Hell' is the way to remember how to tackle stairs after your hip replacement but the same principle applies while you are waiting, if stairs are becoming difficult. Lead with your good leg going up as it can tolerate the bend, and lead with your bad one coming down. Use the bannister, and if both hips are painful, try turning slightly in towards the bannister to improve your comfort.
Arms	Arms are useful and the stronger the better if you have a bad hip. Not only will you need good arm strength after you eventually get your operation to manage the crutches efficiently, but it is also worth improving arm tone pre-op. A good reason is to be able to lower yourself down onto the loo more easily as you may not be able to rely on just sitting down normally as your hip becomes stiffer. So do some arm exercises, press-ups if you can, or maybe some light dumbbells. Of course, if you have a bad shoulder as well, that can be a problem and in certain cases it might be worth getting that attended to before undergoing a hip replacement or using crutches may be an issue. Carrying items (shopping bags, grandchildren, etc) inevitably puts more force through the hips. If you carry

	a shopping bag on the *same* side as your bad hip, it will hurt less than if it is in the opposite hand. I won't bore you with the biomechanical reasons for this, but it really is true.
Toilet	If you are having trouble getting on and off the loo, consider getting a toilet surround which is a frame that gives you something to push up against. You can buy them easily online or in shops which specialise in mobility matters. Your local Red Cross may also be able to loan you one
Skin	Good skin care is important as bacterial colonisation of skin creases and crevices, which may not cause an actual infection, can lead to the build-up of resistant strains such as MRSA (methicillin resistant staph aureas) which can subsequently get into a new artificial joint. Swabs of your throat and groin will be taken at the pre-op assessment and if you are carrying MRSA your operation might be delayed while you are being treated for it. It is common sense to say you should bath or shower regularly but do make sure you get to all those crevices and don't let your stiff hip stop you. I have no particular advice about what soap to use but generally try and use simple soaps. It is possible that antiseptic varieties may allow the proliferation of resistant bugs, but I have no evidence for that. Needless to say, you must have any broken skin looked at and managed effectively, especially leg ulcers, as active infection on admission will almost certainly result in your replacement being cancelled.
Feet	Getting down to wash and care for your feet can be difficult as every hip patient will know. The last thing you need while waiting for a hip replacement is a foot infection such as athlete's foot, or an ingrowing toenail. Any active foot infection will be a reason to cancel the operation as there is a risk of bugs getting into the new hip. So, you will have to work on keeping your feet in good shape. I find the stair trick very helpful for nail cutting,

	but if you can afford it, a regular visit to the chiropodist is an alternative. It sounds obvious but washing and drying between your toes must not be avoided just because it's difficult, and you need to find a way. I have a brush with suction cups on the back that sticks to the shower floor, which is very helpful.
Teeth	Active dental infection is a reason for postponement of your operation, and I would strongly recommend seeing your dentist and hygienist well in advance of your likely admission date so that any trouble can be corrected promptly.
Smoking	All smokers know they ought to give up and as an ex-smoker myself I do know how hard that is. But... • Smoking increases your infection risk, • Smoking reduces skin blood flow and can delay healing, • Smoking makes a post-op chest infection more likely, • You won't be able to smoke in hospital and two or three days of that is going to be really difficult, isn't it? Try and give up well in advance. You can tell yourself you will start again once the wound is healed (but by then you hopefully won't want to). Use patches, gum, vapes, hypnotists, acupuncture, or whatever works. Vaping is much less risky than smoking and although it takes a while to get used to, it works for millions of people. And it's much cheaper. And you don't stink of fags.
Alcohol	Moderation is the key (but I'm a doctor so I have to say that don't I?). Let's just say it is sensible to not have an alcoholic drink for 48 hours pre-op, as you don't want any residual alcohol in the system interacting with the opiate painkillers and anaesthetic drugs you may receive during and after the op.
Diet	Attempts at weight-loss notwithstanding, eat sensibly and regularly. It's best if you have a diet that gives you a regular bowel habit and do try to avoid being constipated.

	Opiate-based drugs tend to bung you up and you really don't want to have to struggle with that post-op, particularly as sitting on the loo for any length of time is likely to be uncomfortable.
Kitchen	You might want to consider moving commonly used items out of low drawers and cupboards to avoid having to bend down frequently. Maybe perching on a high stool would help when preparing food?
Sex	I have undertaken several hip replacements in my career, principally because the patients in question found their hip was preventing them either having or enjoying sex. It was not common for that to be the main reason for their referral, but it was in fact why they wanted the operation at that point in their lives. Most couples find a way and I'm not going to go into detail about that, but if the hip stiffness is so bad that it's not possible to find a comfortable position, don't be shy about telling your GP and surgeon.

Keep the faith

I know it's hard and the wait seems interminable. You may spend months hearing nothing from the hospital and you'll wonder if you have been forgotten. Contact your consultant's secretary every now and then – not too often - and they should be able to give you some idea of when your op is likely to go ahead.

Despite the current difficulties, patients will all get their ops eventually. It may be that you are asked to travel or be transferred to another consultant or another hospital. If you are lucky, you might be taken on by a private provider which should mean a single room and better food, although it will be exactly the same hip replacement done in the the same way.

There has been a trend towards going abroad at much less cost than private hospitals in UK. I cannot tell you that is the wrong thing to do but my biggest concern is what if a wheel falls off after you return home and you have a complication? Returning to the hospital in Europe or beyond might not be feasible and although the NHS will always be there for you, there may be more of a delay than there would have been if you had had your op in your local hospital. It's a risk that I, personally, would not take.

Private arrangements

We are seeing a large increase in patients choosing to self-pay for their operations while the current crisis continues. Many providers offer finance at low rates and the quotes do include everything and cover possible complications. Having a hip replacement privately varies around the country and the all-in cost is about £14,000-£16,000 at present. That includes all the fees and there should be no other unexpected invoices once it has been paid. Your operation will be performed by a consultant not a trainee, and the aftercare may be a little more comfortable in a single room.

New car or new hip? Just asking.

Also, if you are thinking of who to see about having a hip replacement, how do you choose? GPs usually know who is good, both technically, and who has a pleasant 'bedside manner' and takes care of their patients. If you were thinking of having a new kitchen or a new roof, let's say, you might ask around your family, neighbours and friends to get a feel for who has a good reputation. The same applies with surgeons and hospitals, and generally people just know. There is considerable regulation governing surgeons' performance and The National Joint Registry includes individual surgeon data, including revision rates and outcome scores, so that can be a useful source of information.

A cautionary word on that: some surgeons do rather shy away from complex cases, leaving their more adventurous colleagues to take these on – inevitably those more daring operators might end up with a slightly higher complication rate, so don't necessarily take the bald figures as gospel, as there may be more to it.

FINAL THOUGHTS

Hip replacement is arguably the most effective surgical intervention there has ever been. 80,000 are done annually in UK and 90-95% of patients report a good or excellent outcome. 80% or more of modern hip replacements will last in excess of 20 years.

Having had one myself, I can confirm that they really work and do give you your life back. Ignoring the fact that I need the other one doing and am choosing to delay it, my new hip functions perfectly and I never have to think about it. OK, I can't run now, but like Forest Gump, I am finished with all that anyway.

I hope this little book offers you some reassurance and guidance while you are waiting and wish you the best possible outcome when you do finally get your date.

Finally, if anyone reading this is in any way concerned that *my* bad hip may be adversely affecting my abilities in the operating theatre, it really doesn't.

And if it starts to, please rest assured that I'll stop and get it done.

ACKNOWLEDGEMENTS

Charlie, my daughter and publisher, as creator of Magic Daisy Publishing, has been fantastic as ever and together with Tobias has proof-read and edited my useless English.

Many thanks to Rich for doing the exercise line drawings for me again. He really should do more arty stuff I think.

My wife Lorraine has patiently endured my self-imposed wait just as much as I have. She has been robustly practical as always, making sensible suggestions about what I should include in – and what I should leave out of - this little guide.

I am very grateful for the many points I have included which stem from things my patients have told me over the years, and I hope that the vast majority of them would concur that the wait was worth it.

Finally, Fiona Goult has been every bit as supportive with this book as she has always been as a superb physiotherapist over the 20 years we have worked together - especially when *I* was the patient in 2021. I am most grateful for her input to the Exercise and Tips sections in particular, and I am certain that *Waiting for a new hip?* has vastly more credibility as a result.

Also available by Jonathan Hull from Amazon.co.uk &
magicdaisy.co.uk:

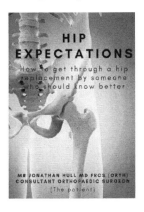

*'Friendly and humorous, expert but not bossy, practical without being
unrealistic' - Michelle (pre-op patient)*
Jonathan's account of his own operation and recovery. Over 500 copies
sold. 4.7/5.0 rating on Amazon. £6.99

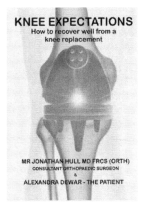

*'...it doesn't put you off the operation, but with his humour, makes you feel
ready for the "ordeal"'- Martin (post-op patient)*
Jonathan and Alexandra describe her experience and recovery following her
knee replacement. 5.0/5.0 rating on Amazon. £6.99

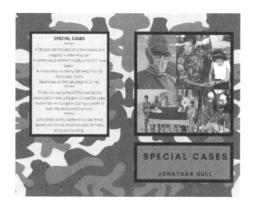

'Funny, sad and fascinating all in one book. Jonathan's style of writing is
what I'd describe as easy, enjoyable reading' - Amazon review
This collection of bizarre but totally true case stories from Jonathan's 40
year career in both the Army and the NHS will amaze, amuse and shock you.
Not for the faint-hearted! Amazon. £8.99

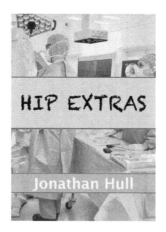

A guide to the things that can spoil a good outcome after hip surgery,
and what can be done about them.
Independently published. Available from jonathanh@jointreaction.co.uk.
£4.99

Magic Daisy Publishing is an independent imprint which supports authors and illustrators who are interested in becoming published.

We'd love you to check out our website:

www.magicdaisypublishing.co.uk

If you have any feedback or would like to get in touch then you can email us:

magicdaisypublishing@outlook.com

You can also find us on Facebook where we have more information about our authors, illustrators and future competitions.

www.facebook.com/magicdaisypublishing

Thank you for your interest in Magic Daisy Publishing!

Printed in Great Britain
by Amazon

33666077R00031